I0560446

From Cheers To Tears

THE REAL IMPACT OF DRINKING

GEORGE J HATCHER

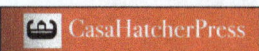
CasaHatcherPress

Dedication

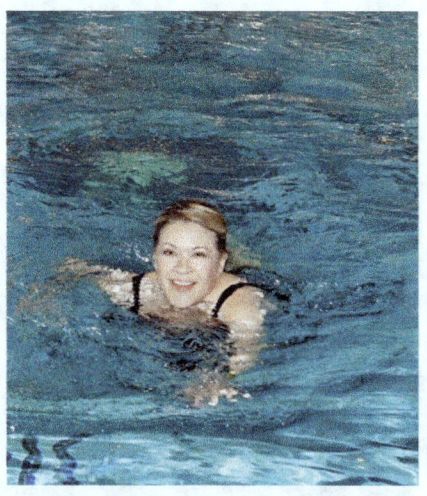

Molly,

In the dance of life, you are my steady partner,

and in every melody, you are my cherished harmony.

With enduring love,

George

This book can be purchased at over 40,000 bookstores and libraries including brick and mortar stores, online, in print and digital, including Apple, Kindle, and Audible formats. Casa Hatcher Press is a subsidiary of Pretty Face, Inc. Rancho Mirage, California 92270.

Casa Hatcher Press. http://casahatcherpress.com (800) 416-6189

Copyright © 2025 by George Hatcher. All rights reserved. Printed in the United States of America and abroad.

No part of this book may be used in any manner except in the case of brief quotations in critical articles or reviews.

Book and cover designed by Casa Hatcher Press

From Cheers To Tears: The Real Impact Of Drinking, by George Hatcher

First Edition June 2025

ISBN: 979-8-9989967-4-0 (Paperback)

ISBN: 979-8-9989967-3-3 (eBook)

Also By George Hatcher

Mario 1: Woman in Jeopardy

Mario 2: Coming of Age

Mario 3: Risky Business

Mario 4: Free Fall

Mario 5: Afire

Mario 6: Marked

Mario 7: Aftershock

Mario 8: Captivated

Single Titles

One Wilshire

Gabi

Rico

Cats: Meow Is The Language Of Love

HER: Artistic Expressions Through AI

Elegance In White: Through Wedding Gowns

Quinceañera Fashion: Fifteen & Fabulous

Billion Dollar Rainmaker Part I

Pages of Passion Book 1: My First 19 Years

Pages of Passion Book 2: Bold Beginnings

Pages of Passion Book 3: Rising Waves

Beyond The Scale: Health Benefits of Keto for Wellness

Cool Under Pressure: Warm With Humor

Love Is What It Is: Lessons From Everyday Life

Living Fully While We Wait to Die: Mindfulness Amid Mortality

Coming Soon

Pages of Passion Book 5

Pages of Passion Book 6

Pages of Passion Book 7

Mario 9

Gabi 2

Rico 2

Introduction

Introduction: A Personal Journey Beyond the Bottle

Forty years. Four decades have passed since my last sip of alcohol. It's a milestone that still sometimes takes me by surprise, a quiet reminder of a life profoundly changed. Before this long stretch of sobriety, my days were punctuated by the ritual of drinking. The clock hitting five in the evening was my signal, the moment the office technically closed, and the bottle opened. At home, the opportunities to drink were many, and I often took them. I was young, and in those days, I'd say alcohol was my social lubricant; it seemed to unlock a more outgoing version of myself, one that navigated gatherings with an ease I didn't always feel otherwise.

It's important to me to say that my experience with alcohol wasn't one of outward aggression or meanness, a transformation I've sadly witnessed in others. Some people drink, and a hidden, often ugly, part of them surfaces. That wasn't my story. Yet, just because a person drinks, or even drinks regularly as I did, doesn't automatically label them an alcoholic – at least, that's how I've always seen it. Even now, decades sober, every home we've owned has a full bar. Our guests are welcome to enjoy a drink; we've hosted celebrations, like our children's weddings, with multiple bars well-stocked with named brands. My choice not to partake doesn't mean I expect the world around me to abstain.

But the absence of overt negativity didn't mean an absence of consequence. The truth is, there are patches of my younger years, recollections of significant events, even major business decisions, that are frustratingly blank. I was likely drinking, or perhaps battling the fog of a terrible hangover. And hangovers... they were a cruel tax on borrowed joy, a physical and mental toll that became all too familiar.

The turning point wasn't a gentle awakening. It arrived in the stark reality of the 1980s when I was sentenced to prison for white-collar crimes – writing bad checks and my involvement in a scheme that caused a loss to a bank. I took responsibility for my actions and served 42 months. During that time, the choice to drink was removed. Sobriety wasn't an option; it was a circumstance.

Upon my release, the world looked different, and so did my path forward. My wife, who had steadfastly waited for me, laid down a clear line: if my old drinking habits returned, our life together would not continue. Her words carried immense weight. But as I reflect, while her love and resolve were powerful, the deeper reason I didn't pick up a drink again was simpler and more personal: I felt remarkably good. Sobriety, initially forced upon me, had unveiled a clarity and well-being I hadn't realized I was missing. It was a feeling I wanted to keep. This newfound sense of control and health also spurred me to quit smoking cigars and cigarettes, another habit shed after prison.

This book explores the multifaceted relationship many have with alcohol – the allure, the social facades, the hidden costs, and the arduous but rewarding journey to a life beyond the bottle. My story is just one among millions, a personal narrative of finding a different way to live, not out of judgment for those who drink, but from a deep-seated desire for a more present, authentic, and ultimately, a more fulfilling existence. The chapters that follow delve into the complexities of drinking, not from the soapbox of an expert or a counselor, but from a place of shared human experience, hoping to offer perspective and perhaps a flicker of recognition for those questioning their own relationship with alcohol.

The Allure of Alcohol

The Social Facade

In the realm of social interactions, alcohol often serves as a facade, masking deeper emotions and realities. For many drinkers, the initial allure of liquor is tied to the belief that it enhances happiness and fosters connection. However, beneath this surface lies a complex relationship where joy can quickly turn into dependence, and camaraderie can devolve into isolation. This contradiction is a significant aspect of the drinking culture that many find themselves grappling with.

The social facade created by drinking can be deceptive. For those in social settings, alcohol can provide a temporary escape, allowing individuals to feel more confident and outgoing. Yet, this superficial confidence often masks underlying insecurities and emotional struggles. As drinkers navigate social situations, they may rely on liquor to project an image of happiness, even when they feel anything but joyful inside. This dichotomy raises essential questions about authenticity and the true impact of alcohol on social dynamics.

Moreover, the perception of alcohol as a means to happiness can lead to a dangerous cycle. Many drinkers may initially experience a sense of euphoria or relaxation, but as tolerance builds, the same amount of alcohol may no longer suffice to achieve that desired state. This can lead to increased consumption in an attempt to recapture fleeting moments of joy, perpetuating a cycle of dependency that ultimately diminishes genuine happiness and satisfaction in life.

As individuals begin to recognize the limitations of this social facade, the journey toward sobriety can commence. Understanding that true happiness and meaningful connections can exist without alcohol is a powerful revelation. It invites drinkers to explore healthier coping mechanisms and to engage with others in more authentic ways. This transformation is not only about quitting alcohol but also about redefining one's social identity and relationships.

Ultimately, the journey from the facade of social drinking to a life of sobriety is fraught with challenges, yet it is profoundly rewarding. Embracing authenticity over illusion allows individuals to foster genuine connections and rediscover the joy that exists in everyday moments. By peeling back the layers of the social facade, drinkers can cultivate a life marked by clarity, honesty, and true happiness that does not rely on the crutch of alcohol.

The First Sip: A Personal Journey

The first sip of alcohol can feel like a moment of pure joy, a fleeting escape from the chaos of life. For many, that initial taste is associated with celebration, laughter, and the warmth of connection. Yet, as the journey continues, it often transforms into something far more complex. What was once a source of happiness can quickly become a double-edged sword, leading to moments of regret and sorrow that far outweigh the initial thrill.

Reflecting on my own journey, I remember the allure of that first drink. It was a rite of passage, a way to fit in with friends during carefree nights out. The laughter was infectious, and for those brief moments, it felt as though all my worries had vanished. However, the euphoria was short-lived, and soon, I found myself reaching for that same glass not to celebrate but to numb the pain of everyday life.

As time passed, the relationship with alcohol evolved, and I began to question its true impact on my happiness. Was this liquid courage bringing me joy, or was it masking deeper issues? Each sip seemed to offer temporary relief, but the morning always brought clarity, a harsh reminder of the previous night's choices. This cycle of temporary happiness followed by regret became a constant companion on my journey.

The process of reevaluating my relationship with alcohol was not easy. It required confronting uncomfortable truths about what I was seeking in those moments of indulgence. I realized that true happiness could not be found at the bottom of a glass. Instead, it was about finding healthier outlets for stress and connection that did not revolve around drinking.

Ultimately, the first sip can symbolize the beginning of a personal journey toward healing and self-discovery. For those who wish to quit, it serves as a reminder that while alcohol may provide fleeting happiness, it often leads to deeper emotional struggles. Embracing this journey means recognizing the need for change, seeking genuine joy, and allowing oneself to heal from the inside out.

The First Domino: A Dangerous Inheritance

It's Just a Beer: The Lie We Tell Ourselves

It's a scene that feels as normal as a backyard barbecue. A father cracks open a beer on a warm afternoon, and his son, maybe fourteen or fifteen, looks on with curiosity. The dad, wanting to bond and maybe feeling a bit of nostalgia for his own youth, holds out the can. "Go on, have a sip. Time you learned how to handle it." It's not meant with malice. In the father's mind, he's not doing harm; he's sharing a moment. He's teaching his son to be "responsible," to demystify alcohol so it doesn't become some forbidden fruit.

But what the son hears isn't a lesson in responsibility. He hears the sound of a door unlocking. He learns that the rules—the laws, the warnings from teachers—are soft and bendable, especially at home. He learns that the refrigerator, once just a place for milk and leftovers, now holds something he has permission to access. The line has been blurred, and it was blurred by the person he trusts most in the world.

This isn't just a theory; it's a dangerous reality. We, as parents, think we can control the lesson, but we can't control the outcome. Research from the National Institute on Alcohol Abuse and Alcoholism (NIAAA) is clear: when parents give alcohol to their kids, it doesn't prevent future problems. In fact, it's associated with the children starting to drink earlier and binge drinking more often. That single "harmless" beer becomes a silent permission slip for the son to help himself to another when no one is looking, and then another to share with his friends to show how "cool" his dad is. The father thinks he's containing the experience, but he has actually lit the fuse. I've seen it in my own family—the path from that first sanctioned drink to a daily habit can be shorter and more direct than any parent is willing to believe.

The Behavioral Gateway

People talk about "gateway drugs," and it can sound like an after-school special, an exaggeration. But the idea of alcohol as a gateway isn't just a scare tactic; it's about behavior. That first beer is the first domino to fall. It may not chemically create a craving for another substance, but it normalizes the very act of seeking a change in your mental state through a substance. It teaches a young person, whose brain is years away from being fully developed, that intoxication is an acceptable form of recreation.

A study in the *Journal of School Health* confirmed that for young people who end up using multiple substances, alcohol is overwhelmingly the first one they try. It's the entry point. Once the boundary of sobriety is crossed and enjoyed, the logic of seeking a new or stronger feeling becomes easier to justify. With judgment already impaired by that "harmless" beer, the willingness to say "yes" to whatever comes next—be it another drink, a pill, or something else entirely—grows exponentially.

You are laying a behavioral foundation. And for some kids, that foundation leads to a lifelong struggle. You see a son you love, who started with beer in your own home, become a man of 54 who still can't get through a day without a drink. The inheritance you pass down isn't just your name or the color of your eyes; it can also be a pattern, a quiet permission that echoes for decades. And that is a hard, painful truth to face.

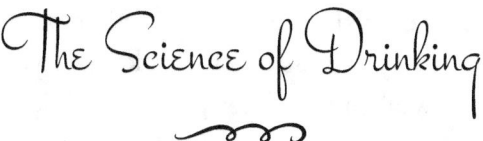

The Science of Drinking

How Alcohol Affects the Brain

When you take a drink, it doesn't just stay in your stomach; it goes on a direct trip to your brain. Initially, it creates those feelings of euphoria and relaxation that we mistake for happiness. But what's really happening is a chemical manipulation, a temporary hijacking of your brain's operating system.

To put it simply, think of your brain as having a gas pedal and a brake pedal. The main brake pedal is a neurotransmitter called GABA, which calms things down. The main gas pedal is a neuro-transmitter called glutamate, which gets things excited and firing. Alcohol cleverly presses down on the brake (GABA), which is why you feel relaxed, less anxious, and sedated. At the same time, it blocks the gas (glutamate), slowing your thinking, impairing your judgment, and affecting your memory. This one-two punch is what leads to that initial "buzz" and, with more drinks, the slurred speech and poor coordination we all recognize.

The problem is that the brain is smart. It knows it's being

suppressed. With chronic drinking, it fights back. It starts to disable its own braking system and slams its foot on the gas pedal, increasing glutamate activity to try and function normally despite the alcohol. This is tolerance. It's why you need more and more alcohol to get the same relaxed feeling you used to.

But this new, rewired state is a trap. When you stop drinking, the alcohol is no longer pressing the brake, but your brain's own braking system is weak, and the gas pedal is still floored. The result is a system in overdrive: anxiety, irritability, restlessness, and the shakes. That isn't just a bad hangover; it's your brain screaming for the substance it has rewired itself to depend on.

The Cycle of Pleasure and Pain

This chemical battle creates a brutal cycle of pleasure and pain. That first drink provides the pleasure—the temporary relief from stress, the boost in a social setting. This immediate reward reinforces the illusion that alcohol is a solution, a key to happiness. But as the alcohol wears off and your over-stimulated brain takes over, the pain arrives. It comes as anxiety, regret, and a general feeling of physical and mental unease.

So, what seems like the most logical solution to this new pain? Another drink. Taking another drink pushes the brake pedal down again, providing relief from the very symptoms the last drink caused. This is the loop that traps so many. You aren't just drinking for pleasure anymore; you are drinking to escape the pain of *not* drinking.

The consequences of this cycle are devastating. Your brain starts to forget how to find pleasure in normal things. A good meal, a conversation with a friend, a beautiful sunset—they don't provide the same chemical rush. The brain's reward system has been re-engineered to respond primarily to alcohol. This is how a habit becomes a dependency, and how the pursuit of a fleeting high leads to a long, downward spiral.

Beyond the Brain: The Body's Silent Toll

While the war is being waged in your brain, the rest of your body is suffering in silence, often with no symptoms until the damage is severe.

Your liver, the body's primary filter, takes the brunt of the abuse. Each time it filters alcohol, some of its own cells die. While the liver can regenerate, with constant, heavy drinking, it can't keep up. The first stage is often "fatty liver," a reversible condition if you stop drinking. But continue, and you risk alcoholic hepatitis—a serious inflammation. From there, the final stage is cirrhosis, where healthy liver tissue is replaced by permanent scar tissue. The liver becomes hard and shrunken, unable to do its job. It's a quiet disease until it's not, ending in jaundice (yellow skin and eyes), internal bleeding, and confusion as toxins build up in your blood.

Your heart is another silent victim. Chronic heavy drinking is toxic to the heart muscle. It can lead to high blood pressure and a condition called alcoholic cardiomyopathy, where the heart muscle weakens, stretches, and can no longer pump blood efficiently. This leads to fatigue, shortness of breath, and swelling in the legs and feet. Essentially, you are poisoning the very engine that keeps you alive.

And then there's sleep. Many people use alcohol as a sleep aid, and it works—at first. It helps you fall asleep because it's a sedative. But it's a trick. Alcohol severely disrupts the most restorative stage of sleep, REM sleep. Your body metabolizes the alcohol halfway through the night, and the rebound effect of your over-stimulated brain kicks in, leading to fragmented, poor-quality sleep. You wake up feeling exhausted, which only increases stress and anxiety, making the desire for a drink the next evening even stronger. It's another vicious cycle: you drink because you're stressed, you sleep poorly because you drink, and you're more stressed because you slept poorly.

The science isn't just academic. It's the blueprint for the physical breakdown that accompanies a life of heavy drinking. It's the explanation for the hangovers, the memory loss, and the slow, silent damage that many don't recognize until it's far too late.

Cheers: The Temporary High

Celebrating Life's Moments

I remember when my wife and I were not even 30 yet, living in a great house we rented in Monterey Park. I was doing well, consulting for a lawyer, and we felt like we were on top of the world. We loved to entertain, and we went all out. We'd send out these cool, creative invites for themed cocktail parties. One month, the card would read, "Join us for a Mai Tai Party," and we'd have all the rums and exotic juices lined up. The next, it would be a "Margarita Party," with blenders whirring and salt-rimmed glasses everywhere. We even threw a "Tropical Itch" party, mastering that specific, potent cocktail for our friends. The theme was never just the gathering; the theme was the drink.

It's a familiar story, and it highlights a central truth for so many of us. Birthdays, weddings, holidays, a big promotion, or just the relief of a Friday afternoon—life is full of moments that call for a celebration. And for most of my life, "celebration" was basically a synonym for "drinking." The pop of a champagne cork or the clinking of glasses was the official sound of happiness. The alcohol wasn't just a part of the party; it was the party—the social glue, the catalyst that was supposed to make a good time even better.

But beneath the surface of these curated parties, the curated cocktails often led to un-curated behavior. I remember one time when the booze influenced a well-respected paralegal, a woman who worked for a very serious law firm, to suddenly undress and take to the diving board of the pool, which was surrounded by dozens of well-dressed party people. Another time, a dear friend of mine, a sharp attorney, walked straight into a sliding glass door he didn't realize was closed, crashing hard. We'd laugh these things off the next day as classic party stories, but they were cracks in the facade. They were moments where the "fun" teetered on the edge of something else—something messy, embarrassing, and even dangerous. It's the price of admission for a party where alcohol is the main event; you never know who is going to pay it, or how.

But there's a catch to celebrating with a substance. Alcohol doesn't actually create joy; it just borrows it from tomorrow. It gives you a loud, blurry, often fragmented version of an event. You remember the laughter, but not always the joke. You remember the dancing, but the conversations are hazy. The focus shifts from the people you are with and the milestone you are marking, to the drink in your hand and the feeling it's giving you. The event itself becomes a backdrop for the act of drinking.

Choosing to celebrate sober felt strange at first. It felt like showing up to a party without the required ticket. But then a shift happens. You start to experience these moments in high definition. The laughter of your daughter on her wedding day, the specific words in a heartfelt toast, the warmth of a hug from an old friend —these things aren't just clear; they are etched into your memory permanently. You are fully present. You are not a passenger along for a boozy ride; you are the driver of your own experience.

Even now, when we host parties, our bars are fully stocked for our guests. I find a different kind of joy in it now. I can watch the evening unfold, appreciate the connections and the energy of the room with a clarity I never had before. There's a profound peace in being the stable center of a celebration, a quiet observer who will remember every detail of the evening long after the last glass is empty. You learn that genuine connection is the real cause for celebration, not the liquid in the glass.

The Emotional Credit Card

The pursuit of happiness is at the core of who we are, but alcohol sells us a cheap, counterfeit version of it. It offers an illusion, a shortcut to feeling good that ultimately leads to a dead end. Relying on alcohol for happiness is like living on a credit card with a brutal interest rate.

When you drink, you get an instant cash advance on positive emotions. Feeling stressed? Here's some quick relaxation. Feeling shy? Here's a dose of liquid courage. Feeling bored? Here's some manufactured excitement. It works in the short term, which is why it's so seductive. But the bill always comes due. The next morning, you pay for that borrowed happiness with interest—in the form of anxiety, physical sickness, shame, and regret. The higher the advance, the more crushing the debt.

Over time, this cycle bankrupts your natural ability to feel joy. It's like eating sugary junk food for every meal. Eventually, a crisp, healthy apple doesn't taste like much. Your palate is destroyed. Similarly, when your brain gets used to the artificial, high-intensity pleasure that alcohol provides, it gets harder and harder to feel genuine satisfaction from simple, everyday things. A walk in the park, a good conversation, pride in a job well done—they all start to feel dull in comparison. Your emotional baseline gets reset to a state of needing that artificial spike just to feel "normal."

Breaking free from this illusion means going through an

emotional withdrawal. It means learning to sit with your actual feelings—the boredom, the anxiety, the sadness—without immediately reaching for a chemical solution. It's about rebuilding your emotional palate from scratch, so you can once again taste the subtle, authentic flavors of a life lived without a filter. It's a slow process, but it's the only way to find a happiness that is truly yours, one that you don't have to pay back with interest the next day.

Tears: The Hidden Costs

~~~

The Emotional Hangover

Everyone talks about the physical hangover—the headache, the nausea. But the emotional hangover is often far worse, and it's something you can't cure with aspirin and a greasy breakfast. It's that 3 AM wake-up call, your heart pounding with a nameless dread. It's the frantic, foggy attempt to piece together the night before, searching for black holes in your memory. It's the shame you feel when you pick up your phone, terrified to see what you might have texted or posted.

This is the state of regret and emotional turmoil that drinking leaves in its wake. It's a self-inflicted wound. The alcohol that was supposed to numb the pain or silence the anxiety only amplifies it in the light of day. You drink to escape your feelings, only to wake up trapped in a far more intense prison of them.

This cycle is exhausting. It chips away at your self-respect, one regrettable morning at a time. The fleeting moments of a "good time" are paid for with hours or days of guilt and self-loathing. You start to question your own character, wondering who that person was the night before. You promise yourself, "never again," but the promise is fragile because the underlying reason you drank is still there. This turmoil isn't just a side effect; for many, it becomes the main feature of their relationship with alcohol.

The Erosion of Trust

The highest cost of a drinking life is rarely paid in dollars, but in relationships. Trust is the foundation of any meaningful connection, and chronic drinking is like a slow, constant acid rain on that foundation. It begins with small things: a broken promise to be home on time, a dinner engagement ruined by one too many "pre-game" drinks, a conversation you don't remember having with your spouse.

Each incident seems minor on its own, but they accumulate. Your loved ones learn not to count on you. They start walking on eggshells, trying to predict your mood based on how much you've had to drink. Their conversations become guarded, and their plans are always made with a "Plan B" in case your drinking gets in the way. They stop trusting your word, not because you are a liar, but because the alcohol is an unpredictable third party in your relationship.

The person drinking is often the last to see this. You feel like you're fine, that everyone is overreacting. But you can't see the look in your child's eyes when you're slurring your words, or the deep sigh from your partner as you pour another glass. You can't feel the vibrant, happy energy of a room drain away when your mood turns sour. This erosion of trust is the definition of isolation. You can be in a house full of people who love you and be completely, utterly alone, separated by a wall of glass that alcohol has built.

. . .

The Price on Your Livelihood

The business world and the drinking world often go hand-in-hand, but it's a dangerous partnership. I know this from personal experience. Your judgment is one of your greatest assets, and alcohol systematically destroys it. It's not just about the major decisions you might make while intoxicated; it's about the thousand small ways it compromises you. It's the morning you come in too hungover to think clearly, the client meeting you aren't sharp enough for, the opportunity you miss because your mind is foggy.

And then there's the ultimate price. My life is a testament to the fact that bad choices, fueled by the arrogance and poor judgment that can come with drinking, have consequences that can cost you everything. It can lead you down a path where you commit white-collar crimes—writing bad checks, aiding and abetting fraud—things you would never do with a clear mind and a steady moral compass. You can lose your business, your reputation, and your freedom. I took responsibility for my actions, and that meant serving 42 months in prison. There is no clearer "hidden cost" than the sound of a cell door closing behind you. That is the final bill for a life where alcohol was in the driver's seat.

The Ultimate Price: A Knock on the Door

For some, the cost is even more sudden and absolute. We talked about how alcohol becomes a gateway for teens, but when you combine that with a driver's license, you create a weapon of mass destruction. Every year, thousands of families get a knock on the door in the middle of the night and learn that the child they love is never coming home.

According to the NHTSA, nearly one-third of young drivers

aged 15-20 who are killed in crashes have been drinking. They didn't set out to harm anyone. They were just kids, making a bad decision that their alcohol-impaired brains couldn't prevent. They got behind the wheel, and in an instant, they either ended their own life or took the life of an innocent stranger. This is the cost that can't be rebuilt, the debt that can never be repaid. It's the tragic, final destination on a journey that might have started with just one "harmless" beer.

Relationships and Drinking

The Unspoken Roles: Enabler, Hero, and Lost Child

When alcohol becomes a central character in a family, everyone is forced to take on a role to cope with the chaos. These aren't roles you audition for; they are assigned by the silent, powerful force of addiction. The person drinking is the star of this drama, but the supporting cast is just as important, and their roles are just as damaging.

Often, the person closest to the drinker becomes **The Enabler.** This is usually a spouse or a parent who, out of love or fear, shields the drinker from the consequences of their actions. They call in sick for them at work after a binge. They lie to friends and family to cover up embarrassing behavior. They clean up the messes. They believe they are helping, but they are actually building a padded room around the drinker, ensuring they never have to face the hard reality of their problem. They become the primary caretaker of the addiction itself.

Then there are the children, who adapt in other ways. One

might become **The Hero**—the straight-A student, the star athlete, the overachiever. This child's mission is to bring positive attention to the family, to prove to the outside world that everything is okay. They carry the weight of the family's self-worth on their small shoulders.

Another child might become **The Scapegoat**. This is the one who is always in trouble, the one who acts out. Their behavior draws all the negative attention, effectively distracting everyone from the drinker's problem. It's easier for a family to focus on a rebellious teenager than on a parent's out-of-control drinking.

And then there's **The Lost Child**, the quiet one. This child learns that the best way to survive is to be invisible. They don't cause trouble, but they don't ask for anything either. They retreat into a world of books or solitude, taking up as little space as possible. Their needs are buried, and they often grow into adults who have trouble forming connections because they were taught that their presence was a burden.

These roles are a desperate attempt to bring stability to an unstable world. But in reality, they just allow the dysfunction to continue, sometimes for generations.

The Loneliest Crowd: Drinking in a Partnership

There is a special kind of loneliness that comes from being with someone who is drinking. You can be sitting across the dinner table from your partner, but they aren't really there. You are talking to them, but the conversation is one-sided, filtered through the haze of alcohol. Their responses are a little too loud, or a little too slow. The person you fell in love with has been replaced by a foggy, unpredictable stranger. The real connection is not between the two of you; it's between them and the glass in their hand.

This is the isolation that a partner feels. It's the silent understanding that their needs will always come second to the need for a drink. It's the heartbreak of knowing that the person they rely on is, in fact, unreliable.

When my wife told me she would leave if I started drinking again after prison, it wasn't just a threat. I understand that now. It was an act of self-preservation. It was the cry of a woman who had spent years feeling the profound loneliness of being married to a man who wasn't fully present. She was not just my wife; she had been forced into the role of Enabler, of worrier, of the person who had to hold everything together while I was disappearing into a bottle. She wasn't threatening to leave *me*; she was refusing to spend one more day in a relationship with my addiction. That's a powerful distinction, and it's one that every drinker needs to understand if they hope to save the connections that matter most.

The Turning Point

Hitting Bottom

For every person who stops drinking, there is a moment when the pain of continuing becomes greater than the fear of stopping. This is "hitting bottom." It's not always a dramatic, movie-like collapse. For some, the bottom is a quiet, internal surrender. It's the exhaustion of waking up with the same regret, day after day. It's looking in the mirror and not recognizing the person staring back. It's seeing the genuine fear in your child's eyes when you reach for your keys.

The bottom is simply the place where you can no longer tolerate your own excuses. It's the end of the road. The lies you've told yourself, the rationalizations, the promises to "cut back"—they all fall away, and you are left standing in the stark, undeniable truth of your situation.

For me, bottom wasn't a metaphor. It was a federal courthouse. It was the cold, hard reality of standing before a judge and taking responsibility for the crimes I had committed—for the bad checks, for my role in causing a loss to a bank. It was the humbling process of watching the life and the business I had built crumble because of decisions made in a moral fog I can only attribute to my lifestyle at the time. The finality of a prison sentence was my bottom. There was no one left to blame and nowhere left to run. The facade was gone, and the consequences were real, tangible, and life-altering.

The First Real Choice

The decision to quit drinking often comes in two stages. The first is when the choice is made for you, and the second is when you make it for yourself.

My initial sobriety was not a choice; it was a condition of my incarceration. For 42 months, alcohol was simply not an option. That period of forced abstinence was, in a strange way, a gift. It was a hard reset. It stripped away the daily noise, the temptations, and the habits, and it allowed my body and my brain to detox from the years of abuse. It gave me the space to experience the world with a clarity I hadn't felt since I was a young man. I had no idea how good it could feel to just be... sober.

The second stage—the real decision—came when I was released. I was a free man. I could have walked into any bar and ordered a drink. And the pressure was immense. My wife, who stood by me through it all, made her own position clear: our future together depended on my sobriety. But while that was a powerful motivator, the ultimate choice had to be mine.

I had to weigh the two lives in front of me. One was the life I knew: the temporary release of a drink, the familiar social lubrication, followed by the inevitable hangovers, the memory gaps, and the trail of regret. The other was this new feeling—this clear-headed, stable, and surprisingly peaceful existence I had been forced to discover.

Standing at that crossroads, I made the first real choice of my new life. I chose clarity. I chose the feeling of being present for my wife and my family. I chose to build a future on a solid foundation, not on the shifting sands of alcohol. That decision, made as a free man, was more powerful than any prison sentence. It wasn't about what I was giving up; it was about what I was choosing to reclaim: myself.

The Journey to Sobriety

You Can't Do It Alone (And Why You Shouldn't Want To)

Once you make the decision to quit, a quiet and often terrifying thought follows: "Now what?" The journey to sobriety is not a path you can walk alone. Some of the toughest men I've known have been brought to their knees by addiction, and thinking you can muscle through it with sheer willpower is one of the biggest mistakes you can make.

For many, the answer lies in support groups like Alcoholics Anonymous (AA) or other programs like SMART Recovery. The power of these groups isn't just in the steps or the slogans; it's in the profound human connection. It's the experience of walking into a room full of strangers and hearing your own story, your own secrets, and your own fears come out of someone else's mouth. In that moment, the crushing weight of shame and isolation begins to lift. You realize you are not uniquely broken; you are just one of many fighting the same battle.

But support doesn't look the same for everyone. A formal

group might not be your path. For me, the most powerful and unwavering support came from my wife. Her belief in me was a lifeline, and her refusal to accept my old life was the boundary I needed. For others, it might be a therapist, a trusted friend, a pastor, or a sibling. The method doesn't matter as much as the principle: you need at least one person in your corner to whom you can be brutally honest, someone who can call you out on your nonsense and remind you why you started this journey when you're tempted to forget. Hiding your struggle is what gives it power. Dragging it into the light is how you take that power back.

Winning the Daily Battles

Sobriety isn't won in a single, grand declaration of victory. It's won in a thousand small, daily battles against triggers. A trigger is anything—a person, a place, a feeling, a time of day—that your brain has learned to associate with drinking. And the fight is about deliberately and patiently rewiring those connections.

The five o'clock itch is real. For years, the end of the workday was my signal to drink. When I first quit, that time of day was a minefield. I learned that I couldn't just sit there and fight the urge; I had to replace the old ritual with a new one. In the early days, 5 PM meant it was time for a long walk, a trip to the gym, or tackling a project in the garage. There was no debate. The old habit had to be crowded out by a new one.

And triggers aren't just about places or times. They are emotional. Stress is an obvious one, but boredom, loneliness, and even happiness can be dangerous. Many people relapse when things are going great, out of a misguided desire to celebrate the way they used to. You have to be just as vigilant on your best days as you are on your worst.

One of the most powerful tools I've learned is a simple mental exercise:

"Play the tape forward." When a craving hits, your brain only wants you to remember the pleasure of that first drink. Your job is to force it to watch the rest of the movie. Play the whole tape. See yourself having the second, third, and sixth drink. See the argument you'll have with your spouse. Feel the shame that will be waiting for you tomorrow morning. Picture yourself waking up at 3 AM with a pounding heart and a head full of regret. When you play the tape all the way to the end, that first drink doesn't look so good anymore. You're not depriving yourself of a drink; you're sparing yourself from the inevitable and painful conclusion.

Life Beyond the Bottle

Living Life in High Definition

For a long time, you might think that quitting alcohol means giving up the fun in life, that you are trading a world of color for one of grey. The reality is the exact opposite. Living with alcohol is like watching your life on a blurry, standard-definition television from the last century. Sobriety is like upgrading to 4K high definition.

Suddenly, you experience the world with senses that have been dulled for years. Food has more flavor. The smell of coffee in the morning is sharper. The sound of genuine laughter—your own and others'—is clearer and more musical. You start to notice the small, simple pleasures that were always there but were invisible through the fog of drinking and hangovers. It's a quiet, profound awakening.

This newfound clarity also applies to your emotions. You feel everything more directly, which can be scary at first. There's no chemical filter to numb the sadness or the anxiety. But you also feel joy, gratitude, and love with an intensity and authenticity you had forgotten was possible. You're not just happy because a substance told your brain to be; you are happy because of a genuine experience. You begin to discover who you really are without the crutch of an alcohol-fueled persona. For many of us, we meet our true selves for the very first time, years or even decades after we thought we knew it all.

The Architecture of a New Life

Building a sober life is an active, intentional process. It's not just about what you *don't* do; it's about what you *do*. You are the architect of this new life, and it's built one solid choice at a time.

The new habits you form are the foundation. Waking up on a Saturday morning for an early workout instead of waking up hungover is more than just good for your health; it's a deposit into your self-respect account. Choosing to read a book, tackle a project, or simply sit on the porch and be present with your family instead of pouring a drink is how you prove to yourself, over and over, that you are in control. These actions build a fortress of self-worth that becomes impenetrable to the old temptations.

Your relationships will also change. Sobriety is a great filter. You will find that some friendships, which were built on the shaky ground of shared drinking sessions, will naturally fade away. This can be painful, but it's a necessary pruning. It makes space for deeper, more authentic connections to grow with people who value the real you, not your drinking persona.

This is how you reach a place of true freedom. It's not about hiding from alcohol for the rest of your life. It's about building a life so full, so strong, and so satisfying that alcohol simply becomes irrelevant. It's how I can have a fully stocked bar in my home for my guests without a second thought. It holds no power because the life I have built is infinitely more rewarding than anything in those bottles. You become the gracious host of your own life, deciding what and who to let in, confident that nothing can take away the peace you have so carefully constructed.

Embracing a New Identity

From "Drinker" to Something More

For a long time, whether we admit it or not, "drinker" can become part of our identity. It might be subtle—"I'm a guy who enjoys a good whiskey"—or it might be the central pillar of our social life. We're the fun one, the life of the party, the one who is always ready with a drink in hand. We don't just drink; we are *drinkers*. And letting go of that label can be one of the most unsettling parts of sobriety. If you're not that person anymore, who are you?

The answer is that you get to be something more. You are no longer defined by what you consume. Your identity is no longer tied to a substance in a bottle. You are defined by your actions, your character, your integrity, and the choices you make with a clear head.

This doesn't mean you have to trade one label for another. For many, the label "alcoholic" is a vital part of their recovery. For others, it may not feel right. I never saw myself that way. I was a man who drank too much, made terrible mistakes as a result, and then chose to stop. My new identity is not "alcoholic"; it is simply "George." It is a man who is a husband, a father, a businessman—a man who is sober. The most powerful identity is the one that is authentic to you, the one that is grounded not in a habit or a substance, but in the simple truth of who you have chosen to become.

Markers on the Path: Celebrating a Life Reclaimed

As you walk this new path, it's important to mark the milestones. A month, a year, five years. These aren't just dates on a calendar; they are monuments to the thousands of good decisions you made. They represent every time you played the tape forward, every time you chose a workout over a hangover, and every time you faced a feeling head-on instead of numbing it.

But don't just celebrate the absence of drinking. Celebrate the life you have reclaimed *because* you are not drinking. On your first sobriety anniversary, take the money you would have spent on alcohol all year and do something meaningful with it. Take a trip you've always dreamed of. Buy a piece of furniture for your home. Invest it in your children's future. Make the reward for your hard work tangible. Let it be a physical reminder of the better life you are building.

Over time, you'll notice the milestones change. The most significant one won't be an anniversary. It will be the day you face a major life crisis—a health scare, a financial problem, a family emergency—and you get all the way through it before realizing that the thought of having a drink never once crossed your mind. That is the moment you know the new identity has truly taken root.

Now, after forty years, I don't think of it as four decades of saying "no" to alcohol. I think of it as four decades of saying "yes." I said yes to being a present husband and father. I said yes to clarity, to health, to peace of mind, and to building a life of which I could be proud. That is the real celebration, and it's one that happens every single day.

Moving Forward

Sobriety is a Verb

There is no "cure" for a troubled relationship with alcohol. There is no finish line you cross where the work is officially over. But this is not a pessimistic message; it is a realistic one. The best way to think about sobriety is not as a destination you arrive at, but as an active, ongoing practice. It's not something you *have*; it's something you *do*.

In the beginning, the "doing" is a white-knuckle fight. It's the moment-by-moment struggle against cravings, the constant vigilance, the hard work of building new habits. But over time, the nature of the work changes. The daily battles give way to a state of peaceful confidence. The "doing" becomes less about actively fighting the negative and more about actively nurturing the positive. The work shifts from avoiding a drink to enjoying a sunset, from managing a trigger to being fully present with your family.

You remain vigilant, not out of fear, but out of respect for the power of the thing you left behind. You remain vigilant to protect the beautiful, stable life you have so carefully constructed. Maintaining long-term sobriety is not about living in a state of constant denial; it's about living in a state of constant gratitude for the life you have reclaimed.

Your Story is Your Strength

This book is me sharing my story. It is not the advice of a doctor or a therapist. It is not the work of an expert on addiction. It is simply the testimony of one man who walked a certain path, took responsibility for the damage he caused, and found a different way to live. I share it not because my story is special, but because I believe every story has power.

Addiction thrives in silence and isolation. It grows in the darkness of shame and secrecy. The single most powerful weapon against that darkness is the truth. Sharing your story—your struggles, your turning point, your journey—is how you break the silence. It is how you turn past pain into future purpose.

You may be reading this because you are grappling with your own drinking. You may be reading it because you are watching someone you love struggle. Wherever you are, I encourage you to find the courage to speak your own truth. Start by telling your story, if only to yourself in a private journal. Then, when you are ready, find one person you trust and share it with them.

You cannot imagine the weight that will lift. You will find that your story is not a source of shame, but a source of incredible strength. It is the proof that you have survived. It connects you to others and frees you from the prison of isolation.

Your journey is your own, but you do not have to walk it alone. Speaking your truth is the first step toward a life you may not yet be able to imagine. I know this is true.

I've lived it.

About the Author

George Hatcher is a man who has always believed that the world is full of opportunities waiting for those bold enough to seize them. With a ninth-grade education and a wealth of unique experiences, he has faced the ups and downs of life head-on. At the age of 20, while serving time, George took the initiative to complete the assignments and tests necessary to earn his high school diploma. His own life is a treasure trove of stories waiting to be uncovered.

Over the years, George has enjoyed a diverse career as an entrepreneur, consultant, and strategist. He has served as a peacemaker for athletes and their parents, as well as a crisis management advisor for physicians and attorneys, achieving considerable success in client development and public relations. He is a licensed boxing manager in California, though he currently has no boxers signed.

George has logged over 200,000 air miles annually through business travel and pleasure trips with his wife. However, since the onset of COVID-19 in 2020, his travel has come to a halt. Now, in retirement, George finds that life remains an ongoing adventure. Unfortunately, he is fighting several new battles that he never anticipated, yet he continues to discover something new with each step.

As a passionate storyteller, George has published a dozen books and finds immense joy in writing. With the world opening up again, he has seized the opportunity to immerse himself fully in his literary pursuits. He currently resides in Rancho Mirage, California, with his wife, Molly, his partner for 60 years, and their home is filled with three cats and one macaw named Peaches. Each experience in his life has taught him invaluable lessons about adaptability, perseverance, and a touch of luck. Like the person who hits their head just to feel the pleasure of stopping, George has made his share of mistakes—some more than once. He hopes others can learn from them as he has.

Now devoted entirely to writing, George Hatcher invites others to join him on this remarkable journey, filled with lessons and stories that showcase the beauty of life's unpredictability.

A longer bio is on his website at
http://georgehatcher.com/bio/bio.html

www.ingramcontent.com/pod-product-compliance
Lightning Source LLC
Chambersburg PA
CBHW071351130626
46556CB00005B/2134